Kicking Butts

D1462423

Books published by the American Cancer Society

A Breast Cancer Journey: Your Personal Guidebook, Second Edition

American Cancer Society Consumers Guide to Cancer Drugs, Second Edition, Wilkes and Ades

American Cancer Society's Complementary and Alternative Cancer Methods Handbook

American Cancer Society's Complete Guide to Prostate Cancer, Bostwick et al.

American Cancer Society's Guide to Pain Control: Understanding and Managing Cancer Pain, Revised Edition

Angels & Monsters: A child's eye view of cancer, Murray and Howard

Because...Someone I Love Has Cancer: Kids' Activity Book

Cancer in the Family: Helping Children Cope with a Parent's Illness, Heiney et al.

Cancer: What Causes It, What Doesn't

Caregiving: A Step-By-Step Resource for Caring for the Person with Cancer at Home, Revised Edition, Houts and Bucher

Coming to Terms with Cancer: A Glossary of Cancer-Related Terms, Laughlin

Couples Confronting Cancer: Keeping Your Relationship Strong, Fincannon and Bruss

Crossing Divides: A Couple's Story of Cancer, Hope, and Hiking Montana's Continental Divide, Bischke

Eating Well, Staying Well During and After Cancer, Bloch et al.

Good for You! Reducing Your Risk of Developing Cancer

Healthy Me: A Read-along Coloring & Activity Book, Hawthorne (illustrated by Blyth)

Informed Decisions: The Complete Book of Cancer Diagnosis, Treatment, and Recovery, Second Edition, Eyre, Lange, and Morris

Our Mom Has Cancer, Ackermann and Ackermann

When the Focus Is on Care: Palliative Care and Cancer, Foley et al.

Also by the American Cancer Society

American Cancer Society's Healthy Eating Cookbook: A celebration of food, friends, and healthy living, Third Edition

Celebrate! Healthy Entertaining for Any Occasion

Kids' First Cookbook: Delicious-Nutritious Treats to Make Yourself!

Kicking Butts

Quit Smoking and Take Charge of Your Health

Published by American Cancer Society / Health Content Products
1599 Clifton Road NE, Atlanta, Georgia 30329, USA

Printed in the United States of America
Designed by Mouse Design Studio, Atlanta, Georgia
Cover designed by Elaine Callahan

5 4 3 2   05 06 07 08 09

Library of Congress Cataloging-in-Publication Data

Kicking butts : quit smoking and take charge of your health.
    p. cm.
  Includes index.
  1.   Nicotine   addiction--Treatment. 2.   Smoking   cessation. 3.
Smoking--Health aspects.   I. American Cancer Society. II. Title.

  RA567.K53 2005
  616.86'506--dc22

                                                    2005020602

A Note to the Reader
The information contained in this book is not intended as medical advice and should not be relied upon as a substitute for talking with your doctor. This information may not address all possible actions, precautions, side effects, or interactions. All matters regarding your health require the supervision of a medical doctor who is familiar with your medical needs. For more information, contact your American Cancer Society at 800-ACS-2345 (www.cancer.org).

EDITOR Amy Sproull Brittain • **COPY EDITOR** Anneke Smith • **EDITORIAL REVIEW** Terri Ades, MS, APRN-BC, AOCN • **MANAGING EDITOR** Gianna Marsella, MA • **BOOK PUBLISHING MANAGER** Candace Magee • **SENIOR LEAD, CONTENT** Chuck Westbrook

Table of Contents

Introduction

YOU KNOW CIGARETTES AREN'T GOOD FOR YOU, but there's something about them that keeps you coming back. What is it that keeps you smoking? And what can help you stop?

This book will help you get to know your enemy, the cigarette, and learn what it takes to defeat it. After you're armed with this knowledge, you'll have one of the most important days in your life—the day you quit smoking.

You're Not Alone

Congratulations! Wanting to quit is an important first step. So now what? How do you quit and what should you do to keep from smoking again? Don't worry, we'll get to all of that, a little at a time.

Quitting smoking can be a real challenge, but you don't have to face it alone. We're going to be here every step of the way, pointing out hurdles to quitting and helping you over them. We'll show you lots of ways to help yourself quit.

By reading this book, you're taking control of the dangerous habit that has seeped into your life one puff at a time. Stick with us: We'll help you turn the tables and kick cigarette butts out of your life for good.

And it all begins here!

Know Your Enemy

The worst enemy is one that poses as a friend and fools you into becoming involved with it. This is just what cigarettes do. So why is something so harmful so hard to leave behind? Because powerful weapons keep you attached to cigarettes. Nicotine, peer pressure, habit, routine, and emotions all play a part in keeping you tied to smoking.

But you *can* quit. You're in control. As you understand more clearly why you smoke and how to break the cycle, you're more likely to kick the cigarette habit for good.

Anyone Can Kick the Tobacco Habit

Smokers aren't the only ones who want to kick tobacco out of their lives. People who chew tobacco or smoke cigars or pipes may also want to quit. Most tobacco users smoke cigarettes, so we focus on cigarette smoking in this book. But the information in *Kicking Butts* can help you no matter what type of tobacco you use. It can also help you help a friend or loved one quit using tobacco.

If You've Tried to Quit Before

You may be one of the many people who have tried to quit before. Having some past attempts under your belt can be a big help. Each time you try to quit, you learn what works and doesn't work for you.

We'll help you look at past quit attempts and figure out what worked and what didn't. And we'll help get you ready to face situations like the one when you started smoking again—without smoking this time.

Battle Plans

There is no right way to quit smoking. People are different. They smoke for different reasons and have different reasons for wanting to stop. It may take some trial and error to find the combination of quitting options that's right for you. We'll outline all of your options. No matter which route you choose, all that matters is that it works for you.

Medications like the patch help many people quit. Counseling and support from others help even more. You're most likely to quit for good if you use a combination of methods.

Each year over a million Americans stop smoking forever. You can be one of them. *Kicking Butts* will walk you through each step of quitting smoking.

How *Kicking Butts* Is Organized

In this book we'll guide you through your quitting options, including medication and support. Then you can explore simple ways to cope with stress, face cravings, keep active, and stay determined. The information and worksheets will help guide you through your Quit Day...and your life as a nonsmoker.

Chapter 1: Facing the Challenges of Quitting

Knowing the challenges of stopping smoking and getting ready for them will help as you quit. This chapter helps you learn why you smoke, the advantages of having tried to quit before, and how to overcome any doubts and fears about quitting. You'll be able to review your personal reasons for quitting to pump up your motivation, read about withdrawal symptoms, and make a commitment to quit.

Chapter 2: How to Quit: It's Up to You

Nicotine, an ingredient in tobacco products, can cause cravings in people who stop using tobacco. The withdrawal from nicotine pulls a lot of people back into smoking. You'll be glad to know that there are safe and effective ways to cut down on cravings and gradually break your body's reliance on nicotine. In this chapter, you'll learn about your many options for stop-smoking medications, which help many people kick the habit of smoking for good. You'll also learn about other methods of quitting and choices of support that can help.

Chapter 3: Countdown to Quitting

As you get ready to quit, you'll find suggestions for how to be with friends or loved ones who smoke; ideas for healthy eating, staying active, and coping with stress; and exactly what you can put in your *Bag of Tricks* (page 65) to get you through Quit Day and beyond as a proud nonsmoker.

Chapter 4: Quit Day

This chapter outlines what to concentrate on during your Quit Day and will help you put your plans from previous chapters into motion. It also includes practical ideas for creating a smoke-free environment, facing cravings on Quit Day, and finding activities to keep your mind off smoking.

Chapter 5: Your Smoke-Free Life

Sometimes reminders can keep you focused as you face each day as a nonsmoker. This chapter helps you look to the future so you'll understand how to face tempting situations without smoking and how to learn from cravings. You're no doubt determined to make this quit attempt your last. But Chapter 5 also addresses how to handle a setback if you do smoke after your Quit Day.

A Helping Hand

This section is offered to those who would like to learn how to support a loved one who is trying to quit smoking. It is an easy-to-read list of tips for significant others and friends to keep at hand.

Resource Guide

The American Cancer Society (ACS) offers programs and services for people interested in quitting smoking. You can find overviews of ACS's and other organizations' important resources and contact information in the back of the book.

Facing the Challenges of Quitting

FOR MOST PEOPLE, quitting smoking isn't easy. But don't worry. Together we're going to work through all the challenges of quitting so you'll be prepared to make your quitting experience as simple as possible.

Most people start smoking when they're young and keep smoking because they like it. They may also like the way nicotine affects their bodies, even if they don't know exactly what it does. People may use nicotine to cope with stress or smoke simply out of habit. In time, some smokers come to feel that smoking is part of every aspect of their lives. But the biggest reason most people continue to smoke— whether they realize it or not—is that they've become addicted to the nicotine in tobacco.

Some strong forces may be keeping *you* smoking—nicotine, the habit of smoking, a psychological or emotional attachment to smoking, or all of the above.

Yes, You *Can* Do It

Here's good news you can believe: *You can quit.* Remember, over a million people do it every year. Anyone can do it, and if you plan for the bumps along the way, you can become a nonsmoker.

Nicotine Is a Drug

It may be hard to think of nicotine as a dangerous drug. Everybody knows nicotine products can be bought legally by adults at grocery stores, at corner stores, or even on the Internet. And you can't really see, smell, or taste the drug nicotine, which is found naturally in tobacco. But nicotine is a powerful drug with serious effects.

It's Addictive

The nicotine in cigarette smoke is what causes an addiction to smoking. Smoking isn't always something people continue to do by choice—even if they don't realize they're hooked on the drug. But *nicotine is addicting like heroin and cocaine.* To understand why, take a look at some facts about nicotine and how it tricks your body into thinking it needs it:

- When taken in small amounts, nicotine makes smokers feel good so they want to smoke more.

- Smokers usually become dependent on nicotine and feel withdrawal symptoms when they stop smoking. When people quit and feel bad, they're tempted to begin smoking again.

- Because nicotine affects the chemistry of the brain and central nervous system, smokers may rely on cigarettes to regulate their moods.

As with many addictive drugs, people develop a permanent tolerance to nicotine. This means that when an ex-smoker smokes a cigarette, even years after quitting, it can trigger a nicotine reaction, hooking the person on smoking again. At some point after you quit, you may get overconfident and think you can handle just one cigarette. Well, just one can be enough to send you right back to your old "pal" nicotine for another long-term visit. Since you don't want all your hard work to go to waste, we'll talk in Chapter 3 about exactly how to cope with everyday stresses without smoking.

People who have already quit smoking say eventually *not* smoking feels as natural to them as smoking used to. Like them, you'll be more likely to live a longer, healthier life when you leave cigarettes behind.

How Nicotine Packs Its Punch

Nicotine affects your body in ways you might not expect. It's a greedy drug that wants to be everywhere at once. When you inhale smoke from a cigarette, nicotine goes deep into your lungs, where it's quickly absorbed into your bloodstream and carried to your heart, brain, liver, and spleen. It affects your heart and blood vessels, hormonal system, metabolism, and brain, among other body parts and functions. It also lowers your skin temperature and reduces blood flow in your legs and feet.

Feelin' Good. Nicotine gets to work right away. It reaches your brain only seven seconds after you inhale cigarette smoke. This is the fastest delivery system of any drug—faster than marijuana, heroin, or cocaine. Then it fools your brain into feeling good by replacing other "feel-good" chemicals (like dopamine) that are naturally present in the brain. Tricky, huh? The first dose of nicotine makes you feel awake and alert, and later doses make you feel calm and relaxed.

The Body's Tolerance. When the body takes in nicotine regularly, it is affected by nicotine less and less. In other words, the body builds up a tolerance to nicotine and needs more and more nicotine to feel good. So a smoker craves cigarettes more often and smokes more often to get more nicotine in the blood. Eventually, a smoker reaches a certain nicotine level

ARE YOU ADDICTED TO NICOTINE?

If you answer yes to any of the following questions, you may be physically addicted to nicotine.

- ❏ Do you smoke within ten minutes of waking up each day?

- ❏ Would you still smoke if you were sick in bed most of the day?

- ❏ Do you have a hard time not smoking when you're in a nonsmoking area?

- ❏ When you've quit or tried to quit before, did you feel withdrawal symptoms or cravings?

- ❏ Have you ever smoked a cigarette when you didn't really want to smoke but felt like you *had* to?

If you answered yes to three or more questions, you may have a strong addiction. Being aware of a physical addiction to nicotine will help you plan a way to quit.

and then smokes as much as necessary to keep this level of nicotine in the bloodstream.

Part of the Problem: Withdrawal

In general, nicotine or cotinine (a nicotine by-product) stays in a regular smoker's body for three to four days after a person smokes. If a person has smoked regularly for at least a few weeks and then either stops using tobacco or really cuts down on the amount he or she smokes, the nicotine level in the person's blood lowers and the person's body begins missing its usual hit of nicotine. This can cause the person to automatically reach for a cigarette to raise the nicotine level in the blood. Without knowing it, the person is treating withdrawal symptoms.

Stopping the use of any drug can cause side effects. If you have withdrawal symptoms after you quit smoking, it's because your body is getting used to going without the nicotine it has learned to lean on. So if you feel physically bad for a few days or weeks, it's because your body isn't getting the drug it wants. Withdrawal symptoms are temporary and are a good sign that you're leaving nicotine behind.

Constant Cravings. Cravings can be predictable—you may crave a cigarette when you first wake up, after your first cup of coffee, or whenever you're feeling angry or upset. When you have a craving, you *really* want to smoke. You may be a little distracted by wanting a smoke, or you may feel like you're going to scream if you don't smoke *right now*. You may feel like there's no way you can get through another moment without smoking.

The good news is: You can. If you don't smoke, you'll get over your craving in a few minutes anyway, and without caving in to nicotine's tricks. Cravings can be very powerful, but *cravings will pass whether you smoke a cigarette or not*. Realizing when and why cravings happen can help you talk yourself out of caving in to cravings when you quit smoking.

You May Feel Bad Because You're Being Good. Withdrawal symptoms make stopping smoking really difficult for a lot of people. But not everyone experiences withdrawal symptoms. Those who do might experience any of the following:

- depression
- feelings of frustration and anger
- irritability
- trouble sleeping
- difficulty concentrating
- restlessness
- headache
- tiredness
- increased appetite
- coughing
- cravings
- mood swings
- dizziness
- nervousness

Smokers who get withdrawal symptoms usually feel them within a few hours of the last cigarette smoked. They will feel the strongest symptoms two to three days later. Symptoms can last from a few days to several weeks. Smokers who have withdrawal symptoms cope with side effects for a while and end up feeling better than they ever did when they smoked. There are many ways you can learn to cope with these symptoms (see Chapter 3).

> ### ▶ HOW TO QUIT
>
> Studies have shown that these five steps will help you quit for good. You have the best chance of quitting if you adapt them to your quitting plan and follow them together:
>
> 1. Get ready.
> 2. Get support.
> 3. Learn new skills and behaviors.
> 4. Get medication and use it correctly.
> 5. Be prepared for relapse or difficult situations.

The Magic of Medications. Medications like nicotine replacement therapy and bupropion (Zyban) can help decrease withdrawal symptoms (see Chapter 2). Nicotine replacement like the patch or gum provides your body with regular, small amounts of nicotine and gradually weans you off of it so you don't go through withdrawal. Zyban is a prescription medication that helps many people cope with withdrawal symptoms.

Leaning on Nicotine

Your need for tobacco is probably not only physical. If it were, you could stop smoking, work through any withdrawal symptoms, and never be tempted by cigarettes again. But for the vast majority of smokers, nicotine addiction is only one piece of the puzzle. People turn to cigarettes for many reasons—to adjust their moods, to cope with feelings, or just out of habit.

> **WHY SMOKE?**
>
> Some people rely on cigarettes to help cope with tension, sadness, or just out of habit. Many smokers use tobacco without stopping to think about the reasons why.

As you read this book and consider quitting smoking, you're working toward your goal of being a nonsmoker. Evaluating your smoking patterns will help you begin to figure out the best quitting plan for *you*.

Smoking is as much a mental addiction as it is a physical addiction. Some people reach for a cigarette to deal with anger or frustration or smoke when they feel happy. When these people quit smoking, they may crave cigarettes as soon as they begin to feel these emotions. They may not be comfortable without smoking to distract themselves from their emotions.

In Chapters 3 and 4 we'll help you find whatever helps you get through your vulnerable moments without smoking.

Smoking "Triggers"

Can you count how many cigarettes you smoked today? Most smokers aren't sure how many cigarettes they regularly smoke. Over time, smokers become used to lighting a cigarette at certain times, when they feel a certain way, or when they're with certain people. You may also face regular triggers—situations, places, people, or feelings—that cause you to want to smoke.

When do you reach for a smoke? In the car? At breakfast? Waiting for the train? When you're bored, stressed, or angry? But you haven't *always* smoked while driving, after eating, when you woke up, or when you felt unhappy. You began associating smoking with these situations, and along the way the situation and the smoking became intertwined in your daily routine. Think about when you use cigarettes to get through your daily life. Do you see any patterns? Take the *"Why Test"* at the end of this chapter to discover your own reasons for reaching for a cigarette.

Certain strategies work best for people who rely on cigarettes for relaxation; others will most help smokers who have become used to lighting up so they have something in their hands. In Chapter 2 we'll address ways to stop from smoking those habitual cigarettes and how you can set up a quitting strategy that will work for you.

The Benefits of Your Doubts

In Chapter 3 we will show you specific ways to cope with some common fears about quitting smoking: preventing weight gain, coping with stress, and spending time with friends and loved ones who smoke. We'll help you set up a simple, effective game plan to handle these challenges.

Many smokers also have general fears about quitting smoking. They may be afraid that it will simply be too hard and they'll "fail," or that it's too late to benefit from quitting. People can quit smoking— and improve their health—even when they've smoked two packs a day for 60 years. With a plan and support, anyone can quit.

"It's Too Hard to Quit"

Mark Twain said, "To cease smoking is the easiest thing I ever did. I ought to know, I've done it a thousand times." Maybe you've tried to quit before too. It isn't easy for most people to give up tobacco, even though they have a lot of reasons to quit.

FEAR OF FAILURE

Reports estimate that for nearly 70 percent of smokers, the possibility of failure stops them from trying to quit. If you set up a plan that's right for you and get all the support you can, you'll have the best chance for success. Don't let fear of failure stop you from becoming a nonsmoker.

Let's be realistic. You won't forget about smoking forever just because you throw away your cigarettes and decide to quit. Quitting involves letting go of the habit, physical addiction, and psychological dependence on smoking.

"It's Too Late to Quit"

It's never too late to stop smoking. Whether you're 18 or 80 and whether you've smoked for a short time or a lifetime, quitting smoking will help you. It will improve your short-term and long-term health, fatten your wallet, stop your clothes, hair, car, house, and mouth from smelling like stale smoke, and help those around you stay healthy.

Your body is capable of repairing a lot of the damage caused by years of smoking. Within 20 minutes of your last cigarette, your body begins healing itself.

Quit Smoking for Good

Although everyone wants to quit on the first try, it takes most people more than one try to kick the habit for good. You may be one of those who can do it the first time. But if you're not, *don't give up*. (See Chapter 5 for more information.)

▶ MY MOST RECENT QUIT ATTEMPT

Reviewing your last quit attempt can help you learn how to improve your chances of quitting for good this time.

What worked?

- What kept me from smoking for a time? *(Thinking about your health? Setting an example for your kids?)*
  _____
  _____

- How long did I go without smoking? _____

- Did I feel any improvements? *(In your breathing or stamina? Your wallet? The smell of your clothes?)*
  _____
  _____

What felt good about quitting?

- ❏ I felt healthier.
- ❏ I helped those around me be healthier.
- ❏ I saved money.
- ❏ Cigarettes didn't control me.
- ❏ I didn't smell like smoke.
- ❏ I set a good example.
- ❏ I was proud of myself.
- ❏ Other people were proud of me.

  Other good things: _____
  _____
  _____
  _____

What was hard about quitting?

❑ Dealing with cravings for cigarettes

❑ Not knowing what to do with my hands

❑ Staying quit when others around me were smoking

❑ Not smoking when *(waking up? finishing a meal?)*:_____

❑ Not knowing what to do when *(angry, nervous, or upset?)*:_____

❑ Other difficult things: _____

_____

_____

_____

What situation, emotion, or excuse led you to smoke again?

• Where was I?_____

• What was I doing? _____

• Who was I with? _____

• How was I feeling? _____

If you came across the same situation again, how could you deal with it without smoking?
I could... _____

_____

_____

_____

Throughout this book we'll outline how you can cope with situations like the one in which you smoked again—and the times and places that make you regularly want to smoke now. *You can handle each of them*—without smoking.

If You've Tried to Quit Before

You may wonder why this attempt to quit might be any different. Having tried to quit before can actually help you quit this time.

About 70 percent of smokers say they would like to quit, and 40 percent of smokers actually try to quit each year. Each time you try to quit, you learn what works for you and what doesn't. So you have an advantage this time around if you've tried to stop smoking before. Think of the last time as a trial run.

Call It Quits: Why Do You Want to Quit?

As you consider committing to quit, think about some "flashbulb" reminders. These will become part of *My Quitting Reminders*—quick, powerful reminders that can stop you in your tracks when you have the impulse to smoke.

Post your list of reasons to quit and the quitting reminders you developed above everywhere you used to smoke so you see them. Don't forget the car dashboard, your desk, your bedside table, and the kitchen. Make a deal with yourself that if you feel the urge to smoke, you'll look at your nearby reminders. Promise yourself that you'll stop and reflect on each reason you wrote down when you started this journey. The urge to smoke will probably have lessened by the time you

▶ MY QUITTING REMINDERS

Think about your unique reasons for wanting to stop smoking. What themes can you see? Health? Money? Control? Other things?

Think about what's important to you as you get ready to commit to quit. What is it about smoking that makes you:

- frustrated? *(Not being able to do the things you want to?)* _____
  _____

- angry? *(The money you spend on cigarettes?)*
  _____
  _____

- tired? *(The control cigarettes have over your life?)*
  _____
  _____

- frightened? *(The effects of smoking on your health?)*
  _____
  _____

What might have the power to remind you of your reasons to quit? Write each one down in large print or tape each one on a piece of paper.

- One word *("cancer"? "health"? "future"? "$$$"? your children's names?):* _____
  _____

- One sentence *("I want to stop wasting money"? "Smoking controls my life"? "I want to live to be 85"? "I don't want to be a smoker anymore"?):*
  _____

- One picture *(a photo of grandchildren? a picture of blackened lungs? a photo of the vacation spot where you want to go with money you would have spent on cigarettes?):* _____

  _____

  What will help you forget about smoking as an option? Your quitting reminders will help you remember why you wanted to stop smoking in the first place.

finish reading. Refer to *My Quitting Reminders* as many times a day as you need to to keep yourself from smoking.

Commit to Quit

Quitting smoking is a lot like losing weight. It takes a strong commitment over time to succeed. That's why only you can make the decision to quit smoking. Other people may want you to quit, but the real commitment to quit must come from you.

You're moving right along on your path to quitting smoking! If you are serious about quitting smoking and feel that you'll be ready to quit within the next month, begin making a quitting plan. The first step is scheduling a Quit Day—the day you'll quit smoking.

Make It Official: Schedule Your Quit Day

Once you've decided to quit, make it official by picking a Quit Day. Choose a day in the next month when you don't expect to be under much pressure or facing a big challenge. Life is full of everyday stresses, but only a major change in your life or a tragedy should make you consider putting off your Quit Day.

ARE YOU READY TO COMMIT TO QUIT?

Do you feel ready to take the next step? Find out by answering the following questions:

- Do you believe that you can make an honest attempt at quitting smoking? _____

- Do you think that you could get a smoking-related disease, and does this worry you? _____

- Do you think that the benefits of quitting outweigh the benefits of continuing to smoke?

  _____

- Do you know of someone who has had health problems as a result of smoking? _____

   Answering yes to these issues means you may be ready to make a serious quit attempt.

You might even want to choose a special day like your birthday, your anniversary, or the *Great American Smokeout*®. Each year about 17 million people try to quit for at least a day during the American Cancer Society's *Great American Smokeout* each November. Of these quitters, more than four million still aren't smoking after three months.

Once you've decided on a date, write it down here.

My Quit Day Is: _____

Make a strong, personal commitment to quit on this day.

- Write your Quit Day on your calendar and in this book to cement its "official" status in your mind.

- Tell friends and family about it so you'll be less likely to put it off.

- Consider the date of your Quit Day sacred, and don't let anything change it.

Congratulations! You're on your way! In the next chapter we'll explore choices of how to quit and help you figure out which of them are best suited to your smoking patterns. That'll help you kick butts for good.

Why Do You Smoke?

This quiz can help you understand why you smoke. Once you understand the reasons why you smoke, you'll be able to create a unique plan for quitting smoking.

THE "WHY TEST"

Next to the following statements, mark the number that best describes your own experience. (5 = Always, 4 = Most of the time, 3 = Once in a while, 2 = Rarely, 1 = Never)

_____ **A.** I smoke to keep myself from slowing down.

_____ **B.** Handling a cigarette is part of the enjoyment of smoking it.

_____ **C.** Smoking is pleasant and relaxing.

_____ **D.** I light up a cigarette when I feel angry about something.

_____ **E.** When I am out of cigarettes, it's near-torture until I can get more.

_____ **F.** I smoke automatically, without even being aware of it.

_____**G.** I smoke when people around me are smoking.

_____**H.** I smoke to perk myself up.

_____**I.** Part of my enjoyment of smoking is preparing to light up.

_____**J.** I get pleasure from smoking.

_____**K.** When I feel uncomfortable or upset, I light up a cigarette.

_____**L.** When I'm not smoking a cigarette, I'm very much aware of the fact.

_____**M.** I often light up a cigarette when one is still burning in the ashtray.

_____**N.** I smoke cigarettes with friends when I am having a good time.

_____**O.** When I smoke, part of the enjoyment is watching the smoke as I exhale.

_____**P.** I want a cigarette most often when I am comfortable and relaxed.

_____**Q.** I smoke when I am "blue" and want to take my mind off what's bothering me.

_____**R.** I get a real hunger for a cigarette when I haven't had one in a while.

_____**S.** I've found a cigarette in my mouth and haven't remembered it was there.

_____**T.** I always smoke when I am out with friends at a party, bar, etc.

_____**U.** I always smoke cigarettes to get a lift.

Now Score Yourself

Step 1: Transfer the numbers from the quiz to the scorecard that follows by matching up the letters. For example, take the number you wrote for question A on the quiz and enter it on line A of the scorecard.

Step 2: Add each set of 3 scores on the scorecard to get the total for each different category. For example, to find your score on the "Stimulation" category, add together the scores for questions A, H and U.

The score for each category can range from a low of 3 to a high of 15. A score of 11 or above on any set is high and means that your smoking is probably influenced by that category. A score of 7 or below is low and means that this category is not a primary source of satisfaction to you when you smoke.

"Why Test" scorecard

"It stimulates me." You feel that smoking gives you energy and keeps you going. Think about alternative ways to boost your energy, such as brisk walking or jogging.

_____ A.　　_____ H.　　_____ U.

_____ "Stimulation" **TOTAL**

"I want something in my hand." There are a lot of things you can do with your hands without lighting up a cigarette. Try doodling with a pencil or playing with putty or a fake cigarette.

_____ B.　　_____ I.　　_____ O.

_____ "Handling" **TOTAL**

"It feels good." You get a lot of physical pleasure from smoking. Various forms of exercise or other activities can be effective alternatives.

____ C   ____ J   ____ P

____ "Pleasure/Relaxation" **TOTAL**

"It's a crutch." It can be tough to stop smoking if you find cigarettes comforting in times of stress, but there are many better ways to deal with stress.

____ D   ____ K   ____ Q

____ "Crutch/Tension" **TOTAL**

"I'm hooked." In addition to having a psychological addiction to smoking, you may also be physically addicted to nicotine. It's a hard addiction to break, but it can be done. Talk with your doctor about using nicotine replacement (the gum, patch, inhaler or nasal spray) to control your withdrawal symptoms.

____ E   ____ L   ____ R

____ "Craving/Addiction" **TOTAL**

"It's part of my routine." If cigarettes are merely part of your routine, stopping should be relatively easy. One key to success is being aware of every cigarette you smoke. Keeping a smoking diary and writing down every cigarette is a good way to do this.

____ F   ____ M   ____ S

____ "Habit" **TOTAL**

"I'm a social smoker." You smoke when people around you are smoking and when you are offered cigarettes. It is important for you to avoid these situations until you are confident about being a nonsmoker. If you cannot avoid a situation in which others are smoking, remind them that you are a nonsmoker.

_____ G   _____ N   _____ T

_____ "Social Smoker" **TOTAL**

Now how do I quit?

Hopefully this quiz has given you some insight into the reasons why you smoke. You can use this information to help yourself stop smoking. Talk to your doctor about how to stop and how to stay tobacco-free.

2

How to Quit: It's Up to You

THERE'S NO "RIGHT" WAY to quit smoking. Things that help you may seem silly to others, and those that help other people may not help you. Don't be afraid to try something new or something you hadn't planned to help you quit. The best way to quit is to use the method that works for you.

Remember how powerful nicotine is? Well, it isn't always easy to drop the smoking habit, and most people need some sort of help as they quit. Using support doesn't mean that you're weak or more addicted than most. It just shows that you're smart to use all the resources you can to increase your chances of success.

Nicotine replacement therapy (the patch, gum, nasal spray, and inhaler) and other medications safely help a lot of smokers quit, and organized support from other people increases success rates even more.

Before your Quit Day, you can prepare for success by creating a personal quitting plan and thinking about the support you'll rely on as you quit. That's what we're going to help you do here.

Talk to the Professionals

Ask your doctor about current information, advice, and suggestions for quitting tobacco use. Even if you choose to stop smoking without using prescription medicine, it's a good idea to check with a health care professional before you quit for the following reasons:

- He or she can review your personal health history and offer advice and information about which medications might be right for you.

- He or she can give you tips on quitting and offer follow-up support.

- Health care professionals are usually the first ones to learn about new, effective ways of quitting. They can also help steer you away from unproven or disproven stop-smoking methods.

Don't Chicken Out: Go Cold Turkey

Most smokers quit "cold turkey." That is, they smoke until their Quit Day and then stop all at once. This is the fastest way to quit and, for most people, the most successful way to quit. Gradually cutting down the number of cigarettes you smoke each day usually doesn't work because a lot of people have a hard time giving up those last few cigarettes.

Never Fear, Medications Are Here

Stop-smoking medications can more or less double your chances of quitting for good. Early evidence shows that combining nicotine replacement therapy with bupropion (Zyban, a non-nicotine prescription medication) may be more effective than using either one alone.

QUESTIONS TO ASK THE DOC

Before your Quit Day, set up an appointment to talk to a health care professional. Talk to your doctor about the details of your health, smoking patterns, and past quit attempts, and any concerns you may have. As you prepare for your appointment, consider the following issues:

I want you to be aware of the following health conditions *(include pregnancy if applicable, and mention any medications you are currently taking)*:

_____

_____

_____

Some things that worked and others that didn't during my past quit attempts: _____

_____

_____

_____

My concerns about medication side effects and nicotine withdrawal are: _____

_____

_____

What do I do if I experience side effects? _____

_____

_____

_____

What can you tell me about nicotine replacement and/or bupropion and my smoking patterns? _____

_____

_____

Medications only treat the physical addiction to nicotine. They cut down on withdrawal symptoms, but they don't magically stop you from being faced with your triggers to smoke. That's why it works best to combine stop-smoking medications with other support. Combining them with a stop-smoking program that helps change behavior can increase your chances of successfully quitting smoking.

Using a medication can help *anyone* who is trying to quit. Nicotine replacement therapy and bupropion are safe for most people. If you're pregnant or trying to become pregnant, nursing, under age 18, smoking fewer than ten cigarettes per day, or have a medical condition, talk to your doctor or other health care provider before taking medications. See also *Is nicotine replacement safe for everyone?* on page 39.

Use It: Nicotine Replacement Therapy

Using nicotine replacement therapy instead of smoking allows your body to get a low dose of the nicotine it's used to without the poisons and tar in cigarettes and cigarette smoke. This helps reduce withdrawal symptoms, in turn helping you reduce cravings and adapt to living your daily life without smoking.

Stick It: The Nicotine Patch. Known generically as nicotine transdermal systems, nicotine patches stick to the skin and provide a constant, measured dose of nicotine through the skin. Read the instructions and safety precautions on the package insert before using the patch. The patch is available over the counter.

Some advantages of the nicotine patch include:

- It's easy to use—you only have to remember to replace the patch each day.

- The constant nicotine dosage helps keep you from feeling cravings.

The nicotine in the patch reaches the bloodstream over several hours and continues entering the bloodstream several hours after the patch is removed, so don't smoke within 12 hours of removing the patch.

Several types and different strengths of the patch are available. If you use the step-down method, the patches you use contain less and less nicotine so you'll be weaned off nicotine without experiencing withdrawal symptoms.

▶ **POSSIBLE SIDE EFFECTS:** A mild itching, burning, or tingling at the site of the patch when it is first applied is normal, but should go away within an hour. Try a different brand of patch if your skin continues to be irritated.

The 24-hour patch almost always causes strange effects, including vivid, colorful dreams and difficulty sleeping. If sleep problems don't stop within three or four days, try switching to a 16-hour patch.

If any side effects are severe or continue, talk to your doctor about using a lower dose patch or trying a different form of nicotine replacement.

Chew and Park It: Nicotine Gum. Nicotine gum (nicotine polacrilex) is a fast-acting form of nicotine replacement. For best results, follow the instructions on the package insert. Nicotine gum can be bought over the counter.

Some of the advantages of nicotine gum include:
- It allows you to control when you receive a nicotine dose.

- The gum may be better than the patch for people with sensitive skin.

- The gum can be chewed as needed or on a fixed schedule during the day.

You don't constantly chew nicotine gum like you do other gum. Chew nicotine gum slowly until you notice a peppery taste. Then "park" it against the cheek, chewing it and parking it off and on for about 20 to 30 minutes. Food and drink can affect how well the nicotine is absorbed, so avoid acidic foods and drinks like coffee, juice, and soft drinks for at least 15 minutes before using the gum and while using the gum.

Chewing the gum releases nicotine, which is absorbed through the lining of the mouth. The nicotine in the gum takes a few minutes to reach the brain, so the nicotine "rush" is less intense than with a cigarette. The higher dose of nicotine gum that is available may help heavier smokers.

Nicotine gum may not be the right choice for those with temporomandibular joint disease (TMJ) or for those with dentures or other vulnerable dental work.

A WINNING COMBINATION?

Studies show that combining the nicotine patch and nicotine gum may be effective. Smokers in most of these studies use the nicotine patches routinely and the nicotine gum when they have a craving. Talk to your doctor about dose strength and schedule if you're considering this option.

▶ **POSSIBLE SIDE EFFECTS:** Some possible side effects of nicotine gum are: bad taste, throat irritation, mouth ulcers, hiccups, nausea, jaw discomfort, and racing heartbeat. Talk to your health care professional if you experience ongoing side effects while using nicotine gum.

Follow Your Nose: Nicotine Nasal Spray. Nicotine nasal spray quickly sends nicotine to the bloodstream through the nose. Read the package instructions and safety precautions before using. It is available by prescription only.

Advantages of nicotine nasal spray include:

- It gives immediate relief of withdrawal symptoms.

- It's easy to use.

- Its quick "rush" of nicotine may especially help heavily addicted smokers.

Follow instructions closely to make sure you get the amount of nasal spray you need to fight withdrawal symptoms. If you have asthma, allergies, nasal polyps, or sinus problems, your health care professional may suggest a different form of nicotine replacement.

▶ **POSSIBLE SIDE EFFECTS:** The most common side effects last about one to two weeks and can include the following: nasal irritation, runny nose, watery eyes, sneezing, throat irritation, and coughing. Talk to your health care professional if you experience ongoing side effects while using nicotine nasal spray.

Take a Breath: The Nicotine Inhaler. The nicotine inhaler is a plastic tube about the size of a cigarette with a nicotine cartridge inside. Read the instructions and safety precautions on the package insert before using the inhaler. The nicotine inhaler is available by prescription.

Some advantages of the nicotine inhaler include:

- You can control the amount of nicotine you get when you have an urge to smoke.

- You may be able to satisfy a craving for a hand-to-mouth action by using the nicotine inhaler.

▶ **WHICH NICOTINE REPLACEMENT IS FOR YOU?**

When choosing a type of nicotine replacement, think about which method will best fit your lifestyle and pattern of smoking.

If You're Looking For	You Might Try	Because
An oral substitute	Nicotine gum	Nicotine gum lets you control the timing of your dosage to help control cravings.
Convenience	Nicotine patch	The patch only needs needs to be applied once a day.
Fast effects	Nicotine nasal spray	Nasal spray works quickly when you have a craving.
A simulation of the act of smoking	Nicotine inhaler	Nicotine inhalers let you mimic the use of cigarettes by puffing and holding the inhaler.

When you puff on the inhaler, the cartridge delivers a nicotine vapor to the mouth. One inhaler cartridge contains about the same amount of nicotine found in two cigarettes.

▶ **POSSIBLE SIDE EFFECTS:** Side effects from the inhaler can include coughing or mouth or throat irritation. You may also have an upset stomach. These symptoms should decrease over time. If you have a bronchospastic disease like asthma, talk to a doctor about whether the nicotine inhaler is right for you. Talk to your health care professional if you experience ongoing side effects while using the nicotine inhaler.

Learn the Ropes

Always treat nicotine replacement medications with respect as you would other medications, and make sure to follow package directions carefully. Package inserts describe how to use each product and address special issues and possible side effects. Many companies that make nicotine replacement systems offer support, tips, and safety information on their web sites. Ask your health care provider if you have any questions.

Safety First

Nicotine withdrawal and nicotine replacement therapy side effects. If you don't use enough nicotine replacement, you may experience withdrawal symptoms that make you want to start smoking again. If you use too much, you could make yourself sick or seriously ill. Read the product insert and follow the package directions. Talk to your health care provider about any questions, and let him or her know if you experience side effects.

CANDY-COATING NICOTINE

Some pharmacies in the United States sell products called "nicotine lollipops" and "nicotine lip balm," which they promote as helpful for people who are quitting smoking. These products often contain a product called nicotine salicylate, a form of nicotine that is not approved by the Food and Drug Administration (FDA) for use in quitting smoking. The FDA has warned those who sell nicotine lollipops and lip balm in pharmacies and on the Internet that the products are illegal.

Other similar stop-smoking products may not use nicotine salicylate and may be legal. Nicotine lozenges are also available, but have not been researched enough to determine their safety or how well they work.

All of these products pose a risk to children because they often look like candy.

You might feel some side effects from the nicotine, like headache, nausea, upset stomach, dizziness, or disturbing dreams. All nicotine replacement therapies produce side effects, but they're rarely severe enough that you should stop using the products.

Depending on how much you smoked, you may still experience some withdrawal symptoms when you use nicotine replacement. Many people who have withdrawal symptoms while using nicotine replacement therapy are using too little of the medication for their specific needs. Talk to your health care provider if your craving for cigarettes continues, if you feel irritable, or if you have a hard time concentrating. He or she might increase your nicotine replacement dosage to relieve these symptoms.

Is nicotine replacement safe for everyone? Not everyone can use nicotine replacement. The following people should get medical advice before using any kind of nicotine replacement therapy or bupropion:

- people with heart or circulatory diseases
- people with high blood pressure
- pregnant women
- nursing mothers
- people under the age of 18

> ▶ **NO SMOKING!**
>
> Do *not* use nicotine replacement if you plan to keep smoking or use another tobacco product. It's possible to get an overdose of nicotine. Signs of overdose include headaches, dizziness, upset stomach, vomiting, diarrhea, mental confusion, weakness, or fainting.

If you take any medications, especially drugs for asthma or depression, talk to your doctor. Your medication dose may need to be adjusted because, with or without nicotine replacement, the body changes when you stop smoking.

Keep nicotine replacement products, including those that have been used and thrown away, out of reach of children and pets. Even very small amounts of nicotine can make them seriously ill.

Is nicotine replacement addictive? Some people worry that they'll become addicted to the small amounts of nicotine in the patch or gum. This rarely happens. Most nicotine replacement products are meant to be used for two to three months. To help you gradually taper off the nicotine, you use smaller doses of these products over time.

Prescription Medications Can Help

The Beauty of Bupropion (Zyban). Bupropion, a prescription drug used to treat depression, is also the first non-nicotine medical stop-smoking aid. It's not clear exactly how bupropion helps smokers quit, but some people think it affects the chemicals in the brain related to nicotine cravings.

Some advantages of bupropion:

- Studies show that bupropion can help reduce weight gain.

- Bupropion is safe to use with nicotine replacement therapy.

- In one study, bupropion patients reported fewer withdrawal symptoms like cravings, anger, anxiety, and sadness than a placebo group.

- Smokers begin taking bupropion before quitting smoking, which lessens cravings by getting the body ready before taking away nicotine.

- People who haven't been helped by nicotine replacement therapies may have success with bupropion.

Bupropion is easy to use. You begin taking it two weeks before quitting smoking to make sure it reaches the right levels in your body to be effective, then you

BE CAREFUL

Don't take bupropion if you have a history of seizures, anorexia, bulimia, alcohol or drug use, or head trauma.

- Don't take bupropion with other medications containing bupropion or monoamine oxidase (MAO) inhibitors (drugs that treat mood disorders).

- Tell your doctor if you're taking any vitamins or herbs as well as any of the following drugs that may have serious interactions with bupropion: Tegretol, cimetidine, phenobarbital, Dilantin, MAO inhibitors, L-dopa, or other seizure medicines.

- Tell your doctor if you have liver, heart, or kidney disease, or if you've recently had a heart attack or bouts of chest pain.

- Don't drink alcohol while taking bupropion.

continue taking it for at least seven to twelve weeks after you quit. It is taken regularly to manage cravings: once in the morning and once in the late afternoon. Early evidence suggests that it may be more effective to combine nicotine replacement therapy with bupropion than to use either one on its own. See the *Be Careful* section above for more information.

▶ POSSIBLE SIDE EFFECTS: Some common side effects from bupropion are dry mouth, difficulty sleeping, shakiness, headaches, and a rash. As many as 3 in 1,000 people taking bupropion may have an allergic reaction—like itching, rash, and hives—serious enough for them to need medical attention. Some people may feel more agitated, anxious, and restless, or have trouble sleeping when they begin taking this drug. If these side effects don't go away after a few days, call your health care provider.

"Maybe" Medications. Other medications, like clonidine (a drug used primarily to treat high blood pressure) and nortriptyline (a drug used primarily as an antidepressant), haven't been approved by the FDA for use in quitting smoking, but they have the potential to help people trying to quit smoking. A government panel has recommended that these medications be tried if other drugs have failed. More research needs to be done to determine their effectiveness and specific dosing requirements. Unpleasant side effects are common with these drugs.

Other Ways of Quitting

Some people may look for support in a number of different areas that have not been proven to be clinically effective in helping people stop smoking in the long run.

- In general, *hypnosis* is not very effective alone, but it may be helpful as part of a comprehensive program.

- Most research has found that *acupuncture* is not effective in helping people quit smoking.

- *Motivational rewards* (for example, setting aside money and having it returned to you after a period of not smoking) are not usually successful in the long run.

- The Office of the Surgeon General reports that *aversive smoking strategies*—techniques used to make cigarettes unappealing, like taking a puff every six seconds or so—can be somewhat successful as part of a comprehensive program. But this method can cause serious physical complications.

- Little scientific evidence supports the effectiveness of *over-the-counter products that change the taste of tobacco*, "stop-smoking diets" that curb nicotine cravings, and *combinations of vitamins*.

Some people also use other unproven methods of quitting, like vitamin therapy, herbal preparations, and homeopathic remedies. Others use mechanical devices like special cigarette filters or machines that punch tiny holes in cigarettes, but no scientific evidence supports their effectiveness. Studies show that products that contain lobeline (which contains compounds with effects similar to nicotine's) do not work.

Support Keeps You Going Strong

If you're serious about quitting, medication alone isn't enough. Tobacco users who try to quit without support usually have a harder time staying quit. Research shows that adding social support to medication

▶ **GET ORGANIZED**

Organized support can help you:

- Learn to predict and avoid temptation.
- Create strategies for handling bad moods.
- Make lifestyle changes to reduce stress, improve quality of life, or make you happy.
- Use mental and physical activities to cope with smoking urges.
- Hear others' experiences with and tips for handling stresses, triggers, and cravings.

THE LOWDOWN ON STOP-SMOKING MEDICATIONS

Type of Medication	Prescription Needed?	Dosage
NICOTINE PATCH (transdermal nicotine system)	NO	15–22 mg a day for 4 weeks; may taper to 5–14 mg a day for 4 weeks. Use for 2–5 months. Available as a 16-hour or 24-hour patch.
NICOTINE GUM (nicotine polacrilex)	NO	2 or 4 mg. Use as needed or use 1–2 pieces an hour on a fixed schedule, no more than 20 pieces a day. Taper the dose before stopping use. Use for 1–3 months (no more than 6 months).
NICOTINE NASAL SPRAY	YES	1–2 doses (one spray into each nostril is a dose) an hour. Use for 3 months and gradually taper off (use for a maximum of 6 months).
NICOTINE INHALER	YES	6–16 cartridges per day for 3 months, then taper off for 3 months (use for a maximum of 6 months). 1 cartridge delivers the amount of nicotine found in 2 cigarettes.
ZYBAN (bupropion hydrochloride)	YES	Begin taking one to two weeks before quitting; after quitting, continue for 7–12 weeks or longer.

How to Use	Why to Use	Disadvantages
Apply to skin every day. A constant dose of nicotine is absorbed through the skin.	Easy to use. Few side effects.	Releases nicotine more slowly than other options. Can cause skin irritation. 24-hour patch may cause sleep disturbance.
Chew slowly, then "park" in the cheek. Nicotine is absorbed through the mouth lining.	Convenient. Can use as needed. Nicotine is absorbed within minutes.	Can't eat or drink (except for water) just before, during, or just after use. Talk with your dentist if you have sensitive dental work or jaw problems.
Spray into nose.	Quick nicotine delivery controls sudden cravings.	Nasal and sinus irritation are common. Those with allergies, sinus conditions, or asthma should not use.
Puff on inhaler.	Few side effects. Delivers nicotine as quickly as gum. Can satisfy hand-to-mouth urges.	May cause coughing or mouth or throat irritation. Not for people with asthma or bronchospastic disease.
Take one pill in morning, one in late afternoon.	Easy to use. Few side effects. May be more helpful when used with other nicotine replacement therapy.	May cause dry mouth or sleep disturbance. Do not use if you have seizures/eating disorders, if you are taking Wellbutrin, MAO inhibitors, or other medications that contain bupropion, or if you are pregnant or breast-feeding.

treatment can boost your long-term quitting success. Including either individual or group counseling in your quitting plan is much more effective than no counseling.

With so many quitting support options, it's critical to enlist the support of your doctor and other resources in finding a program or group that suits your needs.

Strength in Numbers

When other people know about your commitment you may be more likely to stick to it and stay focused on your goal.

Stop-smoking programs help smokers recognize and cope with problems that come up during quitting and provide support and encouragement in staying quit. In general, more intense programs have the highest success rates, so look for a program that has the following:

BE AWARE

Not all stop-smoking programs are ethical. Be careful of programs that do the following:

- promise instant, easy success with no effort on your part

- use injections or pills, especially "secret" ingredients

- charge a very high fee—check with the Better Business Bureau if you have doubts

- are not willing to provide references from people who have taken the class

---

- session length: at least twenty to thirty minutes

- number of sessions: at least four to seven

- number of weeks: at least two

Finding Support Groups. Many stop-smoking support groups are free. Others charge a fee. To find stop-smoking groups in your area:

- Call any of the national groups (or their local offices) in the *Resource Guide* at the end of this book.

- Call your local hospitals to find out about stop-smoking groups in your area.

- Look up "Smokers Information and Treatment Centers" in the yellow pages of the phone book.

The Internet has brought millions of people a new world of communication, including some very helpful stop-smoking chat groups and sites. But beware of any group or literature on the Internet that "guarantees" you'll stop smoking.

IN THE COMMUNITY: Some communities have a Nicotine Anonymous (*http://nicotine-anonymous.org*) group that holds regular meetings. This group applies the principles of Alcoholics Anonymous to the addiction of smoking. There is no fee to participate.

The American Cancer Society (ACS; 800-ACS-2345; *http://www.cancer.org*), the American Lung Association (*http://www.lungusa.org*), or your local Health Department often sponsors quit-smoking classes.

A variety of other health-serving organizations and community- and hospital-based groups offer information on how to quit and where to go for help. Support groups are available to provide emotional support, friendship, and understanding.

AT WORK: Call the human resources office where you work; many companies offer information about stop-smoking programs. The ACS's *Great American Smokeout*® is held in many companies each November. If your company has an Employee Assistance Program, its counselors can direct you to community stop-smoking programs. Your employer might even pay for you to attend a program or partially or fully reimburse you.

Call for Help: Telephone Counseling

Through telephone counseling you can talk to a counselor one-on-one about quitting smoking. Telephone counseling services, or Quitlines, are often sponsored by state health departments. A counselor can support you, give you information, answer questions, and even help you come up with a plan that will work for you. Many counselors have backgrounds in counseling and have gone through a training program. Some are ex-smokers.

Quitlines give callers a place to start and the support to move forward each step of the way. A helpful Quitline offers callers:

- someone to turn to so they don't have to quit alone

- a sense of privacy through telephone-based counseling

- one-on-one motivational support throughout the quitting process

- up-to-date cessation information

- free access anytime, day or night

- referrals to local support resources

The ACS offers telephone services for tobacco users interested in quitting. Contact the ACS at 800-ACS-2345 (*http://www.cancer.org*) for more information.

Your Quitting Plan

You may choose to use one or a combination of methods to quit smoking, including self-help classes or counseling, group sessions, nicotine replacement therapy, or other medications.

Think through the most crucial parts of your quitting plan and commit to trying them by writing them down here:

- Will you quit cold turkey or have you opted to taper down? _____

    _____

- If you will use a stop-smoking medication, which one will you use? _____

    _____

    _____

- Will you use any other methods to complement your quit attempt?_____

    _____

    _____

- Will you rely on some type of organized support? What type?_____

    _____

3

Countdown to Quitting

JUST BY DECIDING TO STOP SMOKING you've taken your first step along the path to a smoke-free life. Most people who relapse start smoking within the first week after quitting, when withdrawal symptoms are strongest and their bodies are still dependent on nicotine. Planning carefully will help you through your first big challenge: the beginning of your quit attempt.

Change Your Mind About Smoking

One of the toughest parts of getting ready to quit is changing your mindset about smoking. After your Quit Day, you'll consider smoking absolutely off limits.

Feeling afraid, sad, or angry about quitting is normal. Try to keep in mind your many specific reasons for quitting. Stay strong. Many people who went into their Quit Days with mixed feelings or doubts became nonsmokers. A positive, no-excuses attitude can help you succeed in quitting.

Cope Without a Smoke

You work through challenges every day. When you quit smoking, you'll simply work through daily challenges without smoking. You can help avoid being tempted to smoke when you come across common stresses by getting ready to face them.

Get Ready for Cravings

As soon as you stop using tobacco, nicotine and other tobacco poisons start to leave your body. If you're hooked on nicotine, your body will send your brain a message—through withdrawal symptoms—saying, "Hello, I need nicotine!" In this chapter and the next we'll talk about how to be prepared for some strong cravings so you won't slip up.

The Smokers Around You

You'll be working hard to keep from smoking again, but some of your friends, family, or coworkers may still smoke. The smokers in your life may be worried you'll judge them for continuing to smoke or pester them to stop too. They may wonder how your kicking the habit will affect your time together. They may not be glad you're quitting or may feel uncomfortable helping you quit. And you may not feel right about turning to them for support when you feel tempted to smoke.

For the first few weeks of your quit attempt you may be especially vulnerable to smoking again. Avoid places where others are smoking if you can. Tell yourself it's okay to leave if people start smoking.

The Picture of Health

It's normal to gain a few pounds as nicotine leaves your body. But not everyone gains weight when they quit, and people who do usually gain only five or ten pounds. Some medications that can help you quit smoking may also help prevent those unwanted pounds.

WHY DO PEOPLE GAIN WEIGHT WHEN THEY QUIT SMOKING?

- Nicotine suppresses your appetite.
- Nicotine speeds up the system and makes people burn calories more quickly.
- When nicotine leaves the body, some people retain a few pounds of water weight.
- People often snack more when they quit because they feel bored, angry, lonely, or stressed.
- A smoker is often used to having a cigarette in his or her mouth and may use food as a substitute when quitting.

A small amount of weight gain is really a matter of perspective. It's much worse for your health to continue smoking than it is to gain a few pounds. Smoking causes more than 400,000 deaths each year in the United States. You'd have to gain about 100 to 150 pounds to make your health risks as high as when you smoked.

Eat and Run. You know that quitting smoking is the best thing that you can do for yourself and those around you. While you're quitting, it may be easier to focus on ways to stay healthy than to worry about your weight. Some steps that will help you condition your body before and during the quitting process:

- Start a modest, regular exercise program.
- Drink plenty of fluids.
- Eat fruits and vegetables.
- Limit fat intake.
- Get enough sleep.

Gradually improving your eating habits may be easier than making many changes at once. Changing your eating habits too quickly can add to the stress of quitting smoking.

Sticking to an eating schedule can help you keep extra weight off, since skipping meals and becoming very hungry before eating might cause you to overeat. To keep yourself healthy, eat a variety of low-fat foods and low-calorie snacks instead of high-calorie, high-fat treats. In Chapter 4 you'll read a few other simple tactics for avoiding weight gain.

Hand-to-Mouth. If you feel hungry between meals, drink water or low-calorie drinks or eat sugarless candy and fruit. Stay away from coffee, caffeinated and sugary sodas, and alcohol, all of which can make you want to light up. Before your Quit Day, think about buying or making low-calorie foods for snacking, like:

- sticks of carrots and celery
- other bite-sized portions of vegetables
- lemon or lime water
- coffee-flavored candy
- sugarless gum
- low-fat cottage cheese
- beans
- fruity or herbal teas
- strong mints
- apple slices
- raisins
- rice cakes

- orange sections
- sunflower seeds
- air-popped popcorn
- butterscotch candies
- flavored decaffeinated coffee
- mini candy canes

- pretzels
- licorice
- lemon drops
- lollipops
- ice

Get Physical. To keep fit as you quit, hit the road, the trail, or the gym for some exercise. Try activities like walking, biking, hiking, swimming, running, weight lifting, or exercise classes like aerobics, yoga, spinning, kickboxing, or sculpting. Keeping active for 30 minutes a day three to four times a week will help you get more fit while also remaining smoke-free.

Exercise also helps cut down on stress, which sends many people back to cigarettes again. It can also help you get rid of the temporary blues that some smokers experience when they quit.

You might be able to pump up your motivation for exercising by getting active *before* your Quit Day. That

▶ **WHAT'S THE PLAN OF ATTACK?**

It's a good idea not only to plan what you'll do when a craving hits, but also to practice your strategy before you quit. On your Quit Day, having to spend a long time searching for a substitute for smoking is a recipe for disaster. Have snacks, drinks, and things to fidget with on hand, and keep a list handy of ways to deal with urges.

way you'll feel better sooner, and when you quit you'll already be well on your way to being more fit. If you don't already exercise regularly, check with your doctor before starting an exercise program.

Get a Handle on Stress

Smokers who try to quit but smoke again often mention stress as one of the reasons they end up going back to smoking. Whether at work, at home, or on the road between the two, everyone—smokers and nonsmokers—experiences some pressure or anxiety. Many smokers use nicotine to help them cope.

You can help your body and mind get used to relaxing before Quit Day. Check your community newspaper, library, or bookstore for stress-management classes or self-help books. Plan specific ways to handle stress. Think of things you can do instead of smoking when stress hits, like:

- chew gum
- squeeze a rubber ball
- take a hot shower or bath
- take a five-minute walk
- read a book
- talk it through

Take a Break. You deserve to take time out of your day specifically to relax. Find a few moments to calm your mind and consciously give yourself a break from daily pressures. Find a distraction or call a friend or someone in your support group to talk through any challenges or stress.

Breathe Deeply and Relax. Deep breathing exercises can help you get through a stressful moment without lighting up. Deep abdominal breathing involves breathing from the lower part of the abdomen. Slow rhythmic breathing involves staring at an object or closing your eyes and concentrating on breathing or on a peaceful scene.

If you find yourself in a stressful situation, step away, then take a slow, deep breath for five seconds, hold it in as you count to five, then let it out slowly for five seconds. Doing this for a few minutes can help you slow down and calm down.

Quiet Your Mind. Spiritual practices like prayer and meditation are often helpful parts of drug and alcohol addiction programs and are integral to twelve-step recovery programs. These spiritual principles can be applied to quitting smoking and can help with stress reduction.

Meditation is a way of relaxing the body and calming the mind to create a sense of well-being. A person meditates by concentrating on a pleasant idea or thought, chanting a phrase or special sound (sometimes called a mantra), or focusing on the sound of his or her own breathing. There are many variations, and a person can meditate alone or with an instructor, yoga master, doctor, or mental health professional. Some clinics at major medical centers and local hospitals offer meditation as a form of behavioral medicine.

Get Ready for Quit Day

From now until your Quit Day, consider spending about 30 minutes a day getting your mind, body, home, work, and support group preparations ready.

Focusing and preparing your surroundings and yourself will maximize your chances of quitting.

Drum Up Support

Support can make a big difference as you quit smoking. Informal support from those around you can really help you stay strong.

Set Other People Straight. Tell your family, friends, and coworkers that you're going to quit and ask for their support while you're quitting and after you quit. Explain what a challenge quitting may be and how much help they can be to you.

Tell those around you about your plan to quit. Ask them to help you stay away from cigarettes and to support you in specific ways:

- Please don't smoke in the house.

- Please don't keep cigarettes in the house.

- Please don't smoke in the car.

- Please don't smoke around me.

- Please don't offer me cigarettes.

- Please say no if I ask for a cigarette.

To thank them for their help, you might make a special dinner or treat them to a movie.

Look to former smokers for support, too. They've been through what you're going through and can support you in unique ways when you have a hard time not smoking.

You might want to ask one family member, one coworker, and one friend to serve as your core support group. Ask them to help support you in specific ways.

▶ WHEN I NEED HELP

Ask a few close friends if you can turn to them to talk you out of going back to tobacco. Write down what you think will keep you from smoking and let these people know what support you need. See the example below.

Name: __David___ The type of help I'd like from you is _Remind me that I want to travel with the money I spend on cigarettes each year (over $1,000). Tell me I can get through this challenge without smoking!_

Name _____The type of help I'd like from you from you is _____
_____
_____
_____

Name _____The type of help I'd like from you from you is _____
_____
_____
_____

Name _____The type of help I'd like from you from you is _____
_____
_____
_____

Name _____The type of help I'd like from you from you is _____
_____
_____
_____

Your Danger Zone

Simple daily events like finishing a meal, talking on the phone, driving, or talking with friends can often trigger your urge to smoke. Recognizing many of your smoking triggers will help you resist them.

Steer Clear of Triggers. You learned *why* you reach for a cigarette by taking the *"Why Test"* in Chapter 1. Now think about *when* and *where* you're most vulnerable to smoking. You may want to develop a list of certain people and places that tempt you to smoke and that you could avoid, especially during the first few days.

Resist Temptation. While you quit, you can avoid certain situations when you'll want to smoke. But eventually you'll need to face these situations again, so you'll want to know how to get through your triggers without smoking.

An important part of resisting triggers is separating the smoking habit from your daily routine. You can practice doing this before your Quit Day by putting off smoking a habitual cigarette—a cigarette you're used to smoking when you're in a certain place, at a certain time, or when you're with a certain

(continued on page 62)

> ▶ **TRIAL RUN**
>
> Even if you're going to quit cold turkey, you might want to try to resist the urge to smoke before you officially quit—at first for an hour, then for a morning or an evening, and then for 24 hours. That way before you quit smoking altogether you can figure out how to best deal with the urge to smoke.

▶ BREAK THE LINK

Part of facing your triggers is breaking the link between the trigger and your smoking. Think about the times and places you usually smoke. What could you do instead of smoking when you find yourself in a "danger zone?"

If you usually smoke...   **What can you do instead?**

After lunch
(Plan to eat lunch at local _____
delis and nonsmoking _____
restaurants, or at your desk?) _____

In the car
(Plan to take public _____
transportation or vary your _____
route to work so you're _____
more conscious that you're _____
making a change?) _____

With coworkers
(Plan to take a short walk _____
with a nonsmoking _____
coworker instead?) _____

When drinking alcohol
(Drink a lot of water and _____
other nonalcoholic drinks? _____
Avoiding alcohol for the _____
first few months after _____
quitting will help you quit.) _____

When...

_____   _____
_____   _____
_____   _____
_____   _____

someone. Instead of smoking when you get off work like you usually do, for instance, tell yourself you won't light up the "after work" cigarette until after you get home. The craving will likely have passed by then. Try taking smoking out of the picture when you feel like lighting up a habitual smoke. See the *Break the Link* section on page 61 for more ideas.

Mix It Up a Little. Changing your routine when you first quit can help you stick to a nonsmoking agenda. Rather than smoking when you wake up in the morning, try drinking hot tea or eating breakfast, jumping in the shower first thing, washing your face with cold water, or otherwise shaking up your morning habits a little.

If you usually smoke with your morning coffee, make a point of drinking your coffee in a different place than you did when you smoked. You might drink your coffee standing up, in a different room, or while looking out the window, for example.

Stay Busy: Nonsmoking Activities

Many of the ways you might cope with stress (calling a friend), urges (distraction), or weight gain (exercise) can also help you keep busy and keep your mind off cigarettes.

When you go to a smoke-free place like a movie theater, museum, library, mall or store, or religious service, you won't be able to smoke. You can also stay busy by exercising, walking the dog, playing ball, spending time with other nonsmokers, playing videogames, or calling a friend.

Plan Rewards for Yourself

You deserve to be good to yourself as you quit. Plan to do something fun every day as a reward for not smoking. Whether it's going somewhere, seeing someone, taking time for yourself, or buying something, write each reward on your calendar and treat each reward as an important appointment.

If you're used to rewarding yourself with a cigarette, plan new ways to reward yourself.

• Go fishing.

• Play a new computer game.

• Visit a friend.

• See a new movie or art exhibit.

• Listen to a new CD.

• Take a hot bath or shower and relax.

• Read outside.

• Buy something you've always wanted.

• _____

• _____

• _____

• _____

• _____

• _____

Choose something you really want to do on your Quit Day and write it on your calendar. Plan to go to lunch with nonsmoking friends to celebrate, schedule a dinner date after work, or go on a hike. Keep yourself busy so you aren't thinking about smoking.

The Day before Quit Day

You're almost ready for your Quit Day. You've worked through many of the challenges you might face as you quit. How else can you make the first few days a little easier on yourself?

- Wash your clothes and bedding to get rid of the stale smell of cigarettes, which can linger a long time.

- Do any errands or chores now so you won't have to deal with them later, like paying bills, catching up on a work project, or finishing a chore at home.

- Get a good night's sleep each night this first week so you're well rested.

Reducing a few everyday stresses will help you manage the challenge of quitting.

Think About Tomorrow. Think through the kind of day you'll have tomorrow. Where will you be? What will you be doing? Who will you be with? Imagine what you'll do at every step during the day. What times and situations might make you want to smoke?

It might help to reread your *Break the Link* worksheet on page 61. Practice what you'll say or do when you encounter temptation or stress. Think through simple ways to cope with each situation without smoking.

Get Motivated. Look over *My Quitting Reminders* on pages 20–21 and pause to think about each of your reasons for quitting. Don't forget to post your lists where you expect to need motivation.

Put Out Your Last Cigarette. Before you go to bed, smoke one last cigarette if you need to. Throw away tobacco, lighters, matches, and ashtrays. Make sure you've searched your house, office, car, coat pockets, and purse for stashes. Now get a good night's sleep so you'll be ready for your first day as a nonsmoker.

▶ **GET READY**

Are you and your environment ready for your Quit Day? This checklist will help you review the practical coping ideas in this chapter.

Your *Bag of Tricks*:

What will you put in your *Bag of Tricks*?

❏ nicotine gum, nasal spray, the patch, or inhaler

❏ support group numbers (800-ACS-2345, numbers for members of your personal support group, and/or others)

❏ an encouraging note from a friend or from your child

❏ *My Quitting Reminders* on pages 20–21

❏ *When I Need Help* on page 59

❏ *Break the Link* on page 61

❏ _____

❏ _____

Cravings:

❑ Are you ready to distract yourself from cravings by keeping busy with other activities like walking, playing on the computer, or talking to a friend?

❑ Do you have gum, hard candies, toothpicks, and low-calorie drinks on hand to bite on or drink instead of smoking?

❑ Do you have a headache reliever, throat lozenges, and cough drops handy in case you feel withdrawal symptoms?

❑ Are you ready to delay for ten minutes whenever you feel a craving?

Support:

❑ Do you have stop-smoking medications ready to go?

❑ If you're using bupropion (Zyban), have you been taking it as directed?

❑ Have you joined an organized support group or set up other counseling services (like Quitline support)?

❑ Have you explained what you need to your personal support group members?

❑ Have you asked the smokers in your life not to smoke around you and not to give you cigarettes?

Exercise:

❑ Do you have exercise clothes and shoes ready to go?

- ❏ Have you booked an appointment with yourself each day to exercise?
- ❏ Do you have exercise videos or hand weights on hand?
- ❏ Do you know the local exercise class schedule?
- ❏ Do you know the community swimming pool's hours?

Nonsmoking Surroundings:

- ❏ Do you have a movie schedule handy?
- ❏ Do you know the hours your local museum is open?
- ❏ If you're interested in religious services, do you know where and when they take place?
- ❏ Do you have any errands to do at local shops or the mall?
- ❏ Do you have meals scheduled at nonsmoking restaurants?

Rewards:

- ❏ Do you have music to listen to that makes you happy or relaxed?
- ❏ Have you listed a few things to buy for yourself?
- ❏ Have you found any nonsmoking pool halls?
- ❏ Do you have any new places where you'd like to go?
- ❏ If you'll reward yourself with a massage, have you scheduled it?
- ❏ Do you have a schedule for your favorite sports team's games?

Quit Day

I T'S QUIT DAY! TODAY YOU BECOME a nonsmoker. You may spend most of your time and energy simply *not smoking* today. That's okay. Just hold on through this first day. Each day of not smoking will become easier.

Put Your Plans into Action

Today's the day to follow through with the plans you laid out in Chapter 3. Here's a step-by-step review:

- **Cope with smoking triggers.** If you can't avoid your triggers, rely on the tactics and ideas in the *If You Used to Smoke When...* worksheet on pages 72–74 in this chapter.

- **Relieve stress.** Take a break, breathe deeply, and try meditating or relaxing. Make a special effort to get plenty of rest for the next couple of weeks.

- **Rely on support.** Rely on the support network you set up in Chapter 3. Go to your *When I Need Help* contact sheet on page 59 whenever you need help working through a craving.

- **Find alternatives to smoking.** Occupy your hands by playing with a pencil or a marble. Use oral substi-

▶ QUICK FIXES FOR EVERYDAY CHALLENGES

Relieve Stress

You may need some quick fixes for coping with stress. When you find yourself upset, angry, or anxious and wanting a cigarette, try one or all of the following:

- Take ten deep breaths.
- Take a hot shower or bath.
- Walk or bike around the block and breathe in fresh air.
- Work in the yard.
- Light incense or a candle instead of a cigarette.
- Shoot hoops.
- Stretch fully, bend your spine, and roll your head gently in circles.
- Work out with a punching bag.
- Visualize a soothing situation and let your body go limp.
- Think about consciously slowing down your thoughts and actions and relaxing your body.

Start Moving

Walking and jogging are easy ways to add activity to your day. And you can do them almost anywhere:

- Get off the bus one stop before you usually do and walk.
- Walk or jog with a friend during lunch.
- Run or walk while exercising the dog.
- Walk or jog while pushing your child in a stroller.

> ### Eat Smart
>
> The following "tricks" can help stop you from gaining weight and distract you from smoking:
>
> - Drink a glass of water before eating a meal.
>
> - Reduce your portions.
>
> - Get up from the table as soon as you've finished eating.
>
> - Brush your teeth or use mouthwash immediately after a meal.
>
> - Avoid sugary and fatty food, which can make you want to smoke.

tutions like cinnamon sticks, celery or carrots, or hard candy if you miss the feeling of having something in your mouth.

- **Keep busy.** Hobbies that keep your hands busy and require concentration can help distract you from the urge to smoke. Needlework, woodworking, playing the piano, working a puzzle, playing a video game, or surfing the Internet can also help keep your mind off smoking.

- **Get physical.** Simple ways to become more physically active include gardening, house repairs, mowing the lawn, playing with the kids, cleaning, and taking the stairs instead of the elevator.

- **Eat smart.** Eating small meals throughout the day maintains constant blood sugar levels and helps prevent you from feeling the urge to smoke. Avoid sugary foods, spicy foods, and alcohol. These can trigger a desire for cigarettes.

71

▶ IF YOU USED TO SMOKE WHEN...

Consider the following tactics for getting through triggers without smoking. Feel free to write in any other ideas you have.

If you used to smoke when you talked on the phone:

- Tell yourself "I don't smoke" before picking up the phone.

- Keep a list of your reasons for quitting by the phone and review it.

- Stand if you usually sit while you talk; sit if you usually stand.

- Walk around or straighten the house while you talk.

- Doodle on a scratch pad.

- File your nails.

- Whittle on a piece of wood.

- Fold a sheet of paper into a tiny square, unfold, and repeat.

- Tear a sheet of paper slowly and carefully into tiny pieces.

- _____

- _____

- _____

If you used to smoke at the computer:

- Create a screen saver that says "I'm a nonsmoker."

- Bookmark a stop-smoking web site or bulletin board and visit it often.

- If cigarettes helped you concentrate, keep a paperweight or other object next to the keyboard and focus on it.

- _____

If you used to smoke during work breaks:

- Take your break, but spend it with a nonsmoking friend in a nonsmoking spot.

- Read a newspaper or magazine during your breaks.

- Sit quietly with your eyes closed and take a mini-vacation.

- If you do spend time with smokers, bring your *Bag of Tricks* from page 65.

- _____

- _____

If you used to smoke when you socialized:

- Sit next to the nonsmokers in the group.

- If you usually drink alcohol, drink nonalcoholic drinks at least half the time.

- Get up often and walk around.

- Take deep breaths.

- Chew on a straw or toothpick.

- _____

- _____

If you used to smoke in the car:

- Take the ashtray and lighter out of the car.

- Sing along with your favorite songs.

- Roll down the windows and breathe fresh air.

- Listen to a book on tape.

- _____

- _____

Create a Smoke-Free Environment

As you prepared to quit smoking you got rid of smoking reminders like ashtrays, cigarette stashes, and the smell of stale smoke. Now that it's your Quit Day, you can develop an even cleaner, fresher nonsmoking environment at work and at home.

Ask family members and friends not to smoke in your house or car. Have gum or mints available as an alternative to lighting up. If family members or visitors feel they absolutely must smoke, ask them to smoke outside.

Get Over Smoking

Any withdrawal symptoms you feel are really symptoms of the recovery process. If your body is craving nicotine, it means it's healing.

Most relapses take place the first week after quitting, when withdrawal symptoms are strongest and the body is still dependent on nicotine. Equipping yourself with all the available resources will help you get through this difficult time. Withdrawal symptoms and the urge to smoke will pass whether you smoke or not.

Your Body Is Adjusting

Your body goes through a lot of changes as it gets rid of all the tobacco ingredients it's grown to love. It only makes sense that it's bitter about being deprived, and that it sends you an angry message. That's what withdrawal symptoms are.

If they occur, withdrawal symptoms usually start within a few hours of the last cigarette and peak about 48 to 72 hours later. They can last for a few days to several weeks. After that, your body will begin to forget about nicotine and you'll feel better. Very few people have every withdrawal symptom, and no one ever experiences all of them at once.

You may not have any of these experiences, but if you do, don't worry, it's normal. As your body adjusts to the absence of nicotine, you may experience some combination of these symptoms:

- **Headache:** Your body is adjusting to increased oxygen in your system and less carbon monoxide.

- **Dizziness or lightheadedness:** Your body is receiving more oxygen than it's used to.

- **Constipation:** The intestines will adjust to a lack of nicotine after a short period.

- **Difficulty concentrating:** Your brain takes time to adapt to working without being stimulated by nicotine.

- **Irritability:** Nicotine affects the chemistry of the brain and central nervous system, so it can affect your mood. At first you may feel nervous or touchy. Try exercising—it may help you feel better.

- **Tiredness:** Nicotine is a stimulant, so when you aren't smoking anymore, you may feel tired.

- **Inability to sleep soundly:** Nicotine affects brain wave function, so you may wake up during the night. You may also dream about smoking.

- **Hunger:** You may think the urge you feel to smoke is really a hunger pang.

- **Coughing:** Coughing helps the body get rid of the mucus clogging your lungs.

- **Dry mouth:** When you stop smoking, your body won't produce as much mucus, so your mouth may feel dry.

- **Depression:** Some ex-smokers say that giving up cigarettes is like losing a best friend. Bouts of crying are common. But these sad feelings will pass. Smoking isn't the solution.

You may not feel exactly the same as others do who are quitting. Any of these feelings you experience will go away, so hang in there. Give yourself a chance to get over smoking.

Your Mind May Play Tricks on You

Like a mischievous devil on your shoulder, your mind may come up with rationalizations for smoking— thoughts that seem to make sense at the time but aren't based on facts. If you feel yourself finding reasons why it's okay to smoke, knock that devil off your shoulder. You're a nonsmoker now, and smoking cigarettes is not an option.

MIND GAMES

If you allow yourself to rationalize, or make excuses for, smoking even one cigarette on or after your Quit Day, you're likely to become a regular smoker again. Expect to have the rationalizations below when you feel the withdrawal symptoms shown. That way you'll be ready and able to see through them.

Typical physical withdrawal symptoms	Typical psychological rationalizations
Depression	I'll just have one to get through this rough spot.
Frustration	Today is not a good day; I'll quit tomorrow.
Irritability and anger	It's my only vice.
Trouble sleeping	How bad is smoking, really?
Difficulty concentrating	Uncle Harry smoked all his life and he lived to be over 90.
Restlessness	Air pollution is probably just as bad.
Headache	You've got to die of *something*.
Tiredness	Life is no fun without smoking.
Increased appetite	I'll gain weight if I stop.

As you go through your first few days without smoking, write down any rationalizations as they come up and recognize them for what they are: messages that can trap you into going back to smoking.

Talk to yourself. If you have the urge to smoke, tell yourself "no." Say it out loud. Practice doing this a few times, and listen to yourself. Here are some other pep talks you may want to rely on today and in the days to come to talk yourself out of smoking:

- "I will not smoke today."

- "Other people have quit, and I can too."

- "Smoking is not an option."

- "This craving will pass in a few minutes whether I smoke or not."

- "I am a nonsmoker."

- "I'm too strong to be tied down by smoking."

- "One cigarette does matter."

- "I don't want to let down my friends and family."

- "I'm too tough to give in to a craving."

- "I want to live a long life."

Withdrawal Relief. Time, home remedies, and stop-smoking medicines like those we outlined in Chapter 2 can all make experiencing withdrawal easier. Many people use a combination of these to work through symptoms. Personal care and over-the-counter remedies can also help ease withdrawal pangs.

Pump Up Your Motivation

Remind yourself why you started thinking about quitting, and don't think of giving up cigarettes forever. Just concentrate on one day at a time. Tell yourself, "I won't smoke today."

▶ TO THE RESCUE

Here are some of the most common withdrawal symptoms and ways you might handle them. Feel free to add your own ideas of ways to cope with specific withdrawal symptoms.

Headache
- Take Tylenol or your usual headache reliever.
- Use relaxation techniques.
- _____

Dizziness or lightheadedness
- Close your eyes for a moment and breathe slowly.
- Sit down and rest for a minute.
- _____

Sore throat
- Suck on throat lozenges or hard candies.
- Drink plenty of liquids.
- _____

Cough
- Use cough drops.
- Drink plenty of liquids.
- _____
- _____

Trouble sleeping
- Cut down on caffeine.
- Read a dull book.
- _____
- _____

Depression	• Talk to a friend.
	• Rely on your support group.
	• _____
	• _____
Constipation	• Increase fruit, fiber, and fluid intake.
	• Exercise.
	• _____
Feeling nervous or irritable	• Cut down on caffeine.
	• Breathe deeply.
	• Take warm showers or baths.
	• Use a punching bag.
	• _____
Difficulty concentrating	• Make a "to do" list.
	• Take extra time to get things done.
	• _____

Your Personal Reasons for Quitting

You've posted your *My Quitting Reminders* list from pages 20–21 where you can see it, and you've tucked a copy into your wallet. When you feel vulnerable to smoking again, rely on this list as a reminder of your reasons for quitting. These reasons are the root of your motivation for quitting.

▶ WHAT YOU CAN DO INSTEAD OF SMOKING: A CHEAT SHEET

Use this at-a-glance list to remind yourself of the many ways you can get through the challenges of quitting smoking with success.

Prevent weight gain:
- Brush your teeth after eating.
- Drink cold water.

Manage your mouth:
- Chew gum.
- Eat hard candy.
- Chew on a straw or toothpick.

Keep hands busy:
- Straighten a paper clip.
- Fidget with a straw.
- Play with a small toy.

Cope:
- Take a deep breath.
- Punch a pillow.
- Scream in the shower.
- Talk to a friend.
- Go for a walk or run.

Distract:
- Take a drive.
- Go to a movie.
- Sleep or take a short nap.

Avoid:
- Leave a tempting situation.
- Spend time in nonsmoking spots
- Don't drink alcohol or coffee.

Relax:
- Write to a friend.
- Take a walk.
- Take a bath.
- Watch TV.

Refresh:
- Read.
- Wash your face.
- Exercise.

Encourage:
- Remind yourself: I can do this.
- Remember cravings will pass.
- Remember why you want to quit.

▶ DAILY CHECKLIST

Make copies of this checklist and use them to keep on track every day. And stay alert: People sometimes get cocky and forget about all the tips and tricks they've learned. Check off each item each day to remind yourself of the steps that make quitting possible.

Date: _____

I'll deal with withdrawal:

❏ Nicotine patch—I'm wearing it.

❏ Nicotine gum, nasal spray, or inhaler—I have it handy.

❏ Bupropion (Zyban) or another medicine—I have taken it today.

❏ Home remedies—I have them handy.

I'll make new routines:

❏ I know what I'm going to do in situations when I used to smoke.

❏ Alternatives—I have distractions nearby to keep my hands and mouth busy.

❏ Activities—I'll keep moving and improve my health while not smoking.

I'll watch out for tempting situations by:

❏ Avoiding them—I'll get away from the situation as gracefully as possible.

❏ Altering them—I'll change what I would normally do until the feeling goes away.

❑ Asking the person I'm with to bear with me because I just quit.

In general, I'll:

❑ Rely on my support system.

❑ Turn negative thoughts around so they don't bring me down.

❑ Spend more time with people who don't smoke.

❑ Go easy on myself because this is a big change.

❑ Remind myself of my personal reasons for quitting.

At the end of the day, I'll ask myself:

❑ What went well? I'll do those things again tomorrow.

❑ What needs to improve? I can change it.

❑ What will my day be like tomorrow? I'll be ready for it.

First thing tomorrow, I'll use this checklist again.

The Immediate Benefits of Quitting

Within 12 hours after you have your last cigarette, your body will begin to heal itself. The levels of carbon monoxide and nicotine in your system decrease, and your heart and lungs begin to repair the damage caused by cigarette smoke. Just think: those positive changes are happening in your body right now simply because you're not smoking.

Treat Yourself

It's the end of your Quit Day. Way to go! You've made it a full day without smoking. On page 63 you planned out rewards for yourself. What's the reward you have planned for today? As you enjoy the reward you chose, think to yourself, "I'm really proud of myself for quitting. I deserve this. I'm working hard at being a nonsmoker." Talking to yourself like this may sound silly, but being proud of your hard work isn't. Don't forget to take a minute to think about all you're accomplishing.

5

Your Smoke-Free Life

B Y NOW YOU PROBABLY KNOW that deciding to quit smoking and staying quit are two different things. Not smoking isn't always easy. But it *is* always good for you and will help you live a longer, healthier life. That's why it can help to stay on top of the things that might threaten to get you smoking again.

Your life as a nonsmoker will get easier, as long as you:

- Stay aware of tempting situations.

- Remember to practice the quitting skills you've learned so far.

- Think of yourself as a nonsmoker.

This chapter builds on what you know about coping with challenges and can help you build a healthy and smoke-free lifestyle.

The Habit of Not Smoking

Like any other habit, it takes time for not smoking to become a part of your routine. But unlike most other habits, not smoking also takes some conscious effort and practice.

Remember Your Coping Skills

These are the major coping skills you've learned to use as you fight the urge to smoke. Use at least one when you're tempted by nicotine.

1. **Never forget why you quit smoking.** Go back to your list of reasons for quitting. Look at this list throughout the day—especially when you feel the urge to smoke. Your personal reasons for quitting are also the best reasons to stay a nonsmoker.

2. **Know when you're rationalizing.** We tend to remember the good parts of smoking and forget the reasons we stopped. You may miss smoking, but don't kid yourself that smoking makes your life better. You know more effective ways to cope or celebrate, like taking a walk or talking to friends.

3. **Don't get cocky.** One of the worst things about cigarettes is their ability to snag their victims again. Don't give in to thoughts of *just one*.

4. **Be on the lookout and prepare for triggers.** By now you know which situations, people, and feelings are likely to tempt you to smoke. Keep using the skills that helped you cope in cutting down and quitting.

5. **Keep busy.** Many new ex-smokers have a hard time coping with boredom. Take up a new hobby, clean your closets, or paint the bathroom. Plan to

be busy. Don't sit around waiting for the smoking urge to grab you.

6. **Reward yourself.** Congratulations are in order each time you get through a milestone without smoking. After a week, give yourself a pat on the back and a reward. No matter how you do it, have fun and be good to yourself in some way. It helps to remind yourself that what you are doing is working.

7. **Think positive.** If negative thoughts start to creep in, remind yourself again that you are a non-smoker, that you do not want to smoke, and that you have good reasons for it. Putting yourself down won't help. Positive thinking will.

8. **Relax.** Use breathing exercises to reduce tension. Instead of having a cigarette, take a long, deep breath, count to five, and release it. Repeat until you're calmed down.

9. **Rely on support.** If you're thinking about reaching for a cigarette, reach for help instead. Ask your informal support group to congratulate you as you check off another day, week, and month as a nonsmoker; turn to your formal support group; or call your American Cancer Society at 800-ACS-2345. We're here to support you.

Keep Up Your Guard

People often slip up and smoke again when they're either under extreme stress or while they're having a great time. If they're upset, they may think, "I used to smoke when I felt bad. Maybe a cigarette would make me feel better." Or if they're happy, they may think, "I used to smoke when I was having fun. I bet a cigarette would help me have even more fun. I've been doing so well. I can go back to not smoking again tomorrow. Just one cigarette, just tonight."

If you find yourself rationalizing having a cigarette, stop! Remember, you're a nonsmoker now. That means not one puff! Nicotine is so addictive that it's impossible for most people to be occasional smokers. If you take even one puff off a cigarette, you're likely to start smoking again. The only way to be safe is not to smoke at all.

"When Have I Quit Forever?" The longer you've been a nonsmoker, the better your chances of remaining one. People who haven't smoked for a year have an 85 percent chance of remaining nonsmokers. Those who haven't smoked for five years have a 97 percent chance of staying off cigarettes. But there's never a guarantee that you've quit smoking forever. That's why keeping up your guard is important. People can quit for years, then smoke one cigarette and find themselves smoking regularly again.

When You're Tempted to Smoke

Even though you've made a commitment not to smoke, you'll sometimes be tempted to light up. Being a nonsmoker simply means not letting your cravings for a cigarette cause you to smoke.

Keep your list of reasons to quit in your wallet so you'll always have a copy when you feel the urge to smoke. Promise yourself that before you have a cigarette, you'll read through and consider each of the reasons you started to quit in the first place. Take a break and think for a few moments about all the hard work you've put into staying away from cigarettes.

Learn from Cravings. Instead of acting on your urges to smoke, keep learning from them. After you quit smoking, the urge to smoke often hits at predictable times. The trick is to anticipate those times and find ways to cope with them—without smoking. Think ahead to those times when you may be tempted to smoke, and plan on how you will use alternatives and activities to cope with these situations.

But remember, even if you slip, it doesn't mean an end to the nonsmoking you. It just means that you should figure out what triggered your slip, strengthen your commitment to quitting, and try again.

You've thought a lot about your triggers while reading this book. Don't forget about them now. Review the following sections:

- The "*Why Test*," pages 23–27

- *Break the Link*, page 61

- *If You Used to Smoke When...*, pages 72–74

Regularly remind yourself of your personal triggers and how you plan to cope when you encounter them.

Be Prepared. You can expect and plan for many urges to smoke. But months or even years after you quit, you may feel an unexpected desire to smoke. To get through urges without smoking:

- Review your reasons for quitting and think of all the benefits to your health, your finances, and your family.

- Remind yourself that *there is no such thing as smoking just one cigarette*—or even one puff.

- Ride out the desire to smoke. It will go away whether you smoke or not.

▶ FACE TEMPTATION

For a few months after quitting, not smoking will take some getting used to. If you're ready for situations when you could find yourself being pulled back to tobacco, you'll do fine.

Risky Situation

Times of Crisis

Troubles—like money problems, losing your job, or illness in the family—can bring on a strong urge to smoke.

Times of Celebration

Good times can trip you up just as bad ones can. You may be used to smoking at parties or as a treat when things were going well.

Down Times

You may have relied on cigarettes as your companion when you were lonely, depressed, or bored.

Time with Smokers

It's hard not to smoke when cigarettes are around, and it's even harder not to smoke when others are smoking. Some smokers may try to get you to have "just one."

Think of other times in your life when the urge to smoke will be strong and write them in here. Make a plan for each of them. What will you do? What will you say?

Ways to Handle It without Tobacco

- Say to yourself, "A cigarette won't make this problem go away."

- Take a walk to give yourself a break and some time to think.

- Talk to someone about what you're going through.

- Pass up alcohol for a while. Dance, talk, and drink soda or juice.

- Don't give in to these smokers' thoughts: "I deserve a treat. I'll just smoke one or two tonight."

- Everyone has these moments.

- Do something active like clean out a closet, take a walk, or ride your bike.

- Get back into an old hobby or take up a new one.

- Pick up the phone and call an old friend.

- Spend less time with people who smoke.

- Stay away from smoky environments, like bars.

- Practice saying, "Thanks, I don't smoke."

Handle Stressful Situations. You've quit smoking, and you may be doing fine until—bam!—something stressful happens and you feel as though you have to have a cigarette to calm yourself down.

The steady stream of stress that flows day after day—things like missing the bus, arguing with the kids, facing a deadline at work, or having no milk for coffee—can be the greatest threat to living tobacco-free.

You've already learned many ways to manage stress without smoking. Find those that work for you, and make these methods of coping your new habits rather than falling back on cigarettes. Review the *Get a*

> ### ▶ HANDLE STRESS SO IT WON'T HANDLE YOU
>
> These ideas may calm you down, give you a fresh outlook, and help you stay away from tobacco:
>
> - **Have some fun.** Each day, find something you enjoy doing and make time for it. Build in "down time" for relaxing.
>
> - **Spend time with your support group.** Gravitate toward people who care about you in your new life as a nonsmoker.
>
> - **Take care of yourself.** Try to eat well and get enough sleep. Keeping your body strong makes it easier to handle stress.
>
> - **Get moving.** Research proves that regular exercise improves your mood and calms you down.
>
> - **Try deep breathing.** It's simple, but it works if you need help in a hurry. When you're under stress, you often start to take shallow, rapid breaths without even knowing it.

Handle on Stress section on pages 56–57 to remind yourself of specific coping methods.

Celebrate without Smoking. Many people's smoking urges are linked to eating, celebrating, and drinking. And most people's urges occur when they're around other smokers. Stick to these tips for preventing urges:

- **Eat well without overindulging.** Pigging out can spark a tendency to overindulge on a regular basis.

- **Stretch out meals.** Eating slowly and pausing in between bites will make the meal more satisfying.

- **Keep busy.** Play host or hostess, serve snacks, and greet guests to keep your mind off smoking.

- **Stay away from alcohol.** If you do drink alcohol, always choose a nonalcoholic drink first. Then water down your alcoholic drinks and put plenty of ice in them.

Spend Time with Nonsmoking Friends. When you first quit, it can be too much temptation to spend time with smoking friends. If coffee breaks at work were really smoke breaks, avoid the usual group for a while. If you rejoin them, expect to feel cravings and expect to be offered tobacco. If you can, create nonsmoking times to spend time with friends who smoke.

Chart Your Progress

Think back over your quit attempt so far. Are you having as many withdrawal pangs or cravings as you did at first? How much time do you spend thinking about tobacco now? If you're having cravings for ten minutes or so every couple of hours, think about this: You're doing just fine for 110 minutes of those 120.

Reward Yourself for Reaching Milestones

Reminding yourself of all the milestones you've reached can help inspire you to continue fighting off the smoking habit. Celebrate your first smoke-free week, your first smoke-free month, your first smoke-free birthday, and any other milestone you can think of.

In *Plan Rewards for Yourself*, page 63, and *Treat Yourself*, page 84, you wrote down small ways to reward yourself for not smoking each day. As you look to the rest of your life, can you think of big ways to pay yourself back for stopping smoking? What about redecorating and getting rid of smoke-stained wallpaper and rugs that never lose the smell of stale smoke? Or going on a weekend hiking trip and enjoying your ability to breathe and move more easily?

Daily Rewards *How I can reward myself each day for not smoking*	**Big Rewards** *How I'll reward myself after each smoke-free milestone*
	One month:
	Three months:
	Six months:
	One year:

IF YOU SMOKE AGAIN

If you do smoke a cigarette, don't be discouraged. Almost everyone who has tried to stop smoking has faced this moment of truth. Many give up and go back to smoking regularly, but you don't have to join them. Keep slip-ups in perspective and learn from them.

Rather than using a slip as an excuse to go back to smoking, look at what went wrong and renew your commitment to staying off smoking for good. The difference between a *slip* and a *relapse* is within your control.

- **A small setback doesn't mean you've become a smoker again.** Your very first cigarette didn't make you a smoker, and a small setback doesn't mean you're a smoker again.

- **Don't buy a pack because you've smoked one or two cigarettes.** Remember that you got through several days, or maybe even weeks or months, without a cigarette. This shows that you don't need cigarettes and that you can be a successful quitter.

- **Don't be too hard on yourself.** One slip doesn't mean you're a failure or that you can't be a nonsmoker. Tell yourself, "I'm not going to let all of this effort go to waste. I'm still a nonsmoker!"

- **Learn from experience.** What caused you to smoke? Boredom? Stress? How will you cope with a similar situation in the future?

- **Know and use the coping skills in this book.**
  People who know at least one coping skill are
  more likely to remain nonsmokers than those
  who do not know any.

- **If you think you need professional help with
  quitting, see your doctor.** He or she can provide
  extra motivation for you to stop smoking. Your
  doctor may also prescribe a form of nicotine
  replacement that helps you break your pattern of
  smoking.

  If you've begun smoking again, don't give up!
  Many smokers can expect setbacks or relapses; it's
  a normal part of quitting. Some smokers try to quit
  multiple times before they quit for good. But
  studies show that each time you try to quit, you're
  more likely to succeed.

  Review your past attempts and identify what
  worked and what didn't so you can use your most
  successful strategies again. Any attempt to quit is a
  step in a healthier direction. When you feel ready to
  commit to quit again, review *My Most Recent Quit
  Attempt*, pages 17–18, set a new Quit Day, and
  resolve to make your next attempt your last. No ifs,
  ands, or butts!

Stay Focused on Your Goals

Stopping smoking may be the hardest thing you've ever done, but you're well on your way to staying quit for good.

You've read this book, and you can always come back to it for tips on staying smoke-free for life. Don't leave all of this behind and think you're ready to go it alone. You're getting stronger every day, but everyone who quits can use reminders and refreshers in how to stay motivated. Some important sections to review regularly are: *My Quitting Reminders*, pages 20–21, *If You Used to Smoke When...*, pages 72–74, and *Daily Checklist*, pages 82–83.

You've worked hard to become a nonsmoker. Since you quit, your life expectancy has increased, the food you eat tastes better, your clothes smell better, you've saved money, and you can breathe easier.

Now that you've set yourself free from cigarettes, celebrate all of the time and energy you've invested in the new you. Sit back and catch your breath. You're on the road to a healthier, happier life. You did it!

A Helping Hand

How to Support a Loved One Who's Quitting Smoking

SIGNIFICANT OTHERS AND FRIENDS don't always know how they can help a loved one quit smoking. This handy set of guidelines can help people support someone they care about during a quit attempt. Feel free to copy this list and keep it handy so you can help your loved one.

- Understand that this may be the toughest thing your loved one has ever done.

- Suggest nonsmoking activities you and your loved one can do together.

- Be patient if your loved one is irritable, distracted, or a little down when he or she quits. Smokers may go through withdrawal from the drug nicotine, but withdrawal symptoms are temporary.

- Ask your loved one to rely on you for support if he or she feels the urge to smoke. Make a deal with your loved one that he or she will call you before lighting up.

- Be a walking, running, or exercise class buddy.

- Remind your loved one regularly that you're proud of him or her.

- Celebrate your loved one's nonsmoking milestones with him or her. Ask what you can do to reward your loved one's achievements.

- Remind your loved one of all the benefits to his or her health, wallet, and self-image.

- If you're a smoker, don't smoke around your loved one. Keep cigarettes out of sight and out of reach when your loved one is around.

- Ask your loved one about his or her biggest challenges to staying smoke free—whether during coffee breaks, after lunch, at the end of the workday, or when feeling stress, for example—and offer to check in at those times.

- Be a custom-made support person...ask exactly how you can help keep your loved one on a nonsmoking track.

- Don't nag or make your loved one feel guilty if he or she slips up or struggles with quitting. Support your loved one through challenges or as he or she tries again.

Resource Guide

A variety of organizations offer information on how to quit and where to go for help. If you want to quit smoking and you need help, talk with your health care provider and contact one of the organizations here. Together they can provide you with current information, advice, and suggestions for ending your tobacco use. You may also want to call your state's Department of Health to see if they offer a state-sponsored stop-smoking program.

American Cancer Society Resources

American Cancer Society
Toll-Free: 800-ACS-2345
Web site: *http://www.cancer.org*

The American Cancer Society (ACS) is the nationwide community-based volunteer health organization dedicated to eliminating cancer as a major health problem by preventing cancer, saving lives, and diminishing suffering from cancer through research, education, advocacy, and service. Call 800-ACS-2345 or visit *http://www.cancer.org* to locate your division office for your state or region, or for more information about smoking cessation or cancer-related topics. The publications listed in the front of this book are available for sale through the Society's toll-free number and Web site and include information about general health, cancer, and prevention and early detection.

Self-Help Materials
Materials are available to help you quit smoking, no matter where you are in the process. You can use the materials to learn how to prepare for your quit attempt, develop

strategies to help with cravings, and prevent relapsing once you have quit. Self-help materials offer proven methods that are easy to follow and can keep your motivation high. The American Cancer Society's "Break Away from the Pack" series has been shown to double your chances of quitting successfully. For more information on "Break Away from the Pack" or other self-help materials from the American Cancer Society, call 800-ACS-2345.

Community Resources

The American Cancer Society can tell you about smoking cessation resources in your community. These may include classes, support groups, Internet resources, or medication assistance referrals. It is important to have support from several different sources during your quit attempt, including family, friends, doctors, and cessation professionals. Call 800-ACS-2345 for more details.

Quitlines (Telephone Counseling Programs)

You may be able to use a telephone counseling program, or Quitline, in your area. You can receive quitting strategies and support over the phone, at times that are convenient for you. Quitlines have been proven to double your chances of successfully quitting. Your state may sponsor a Quitline, or you can enroll in the American Cancer Society's Quitline clinical trial.

The Great American Smokeout

The ACS's *Great American Smokeout* is a special day set aside to motivate smokers to quit for a day—and hopefully stay off cigarettes for a lifetime. Through the *Great American Smokeout* and other year-round tobacco cessation programs and services, ACS continues to inform people about the dangers of smoking and tobacco use and to save lives by providing the tools to help users quit. For more information about how to get involved in the *Great American Smokeout* and to learn about tobacco cessation strategies, visit us at *http://www.cancer.org*.

Other Organizations and Resources

The American Cancer Society does not necessarily endorse the agencies, organizations, corporations, and publications represented in this resource guide. This guide is provided for assistance in obtaining information only.

American Lung Association (ALA)

61 Broadway, 6th Floor
New York, NY 10006
Toll-Free: 800-LUNG-USA (800-586-4872)
Phone: 212-315-8700
Fax: 212-265-5642
Web site: *http://www.lungusa.org*

ALA is a voluntary, nonprofit agency fighting lung diseases. Its mission is to prevent lung disease and promote lung health, with special emphasis on asthma, tobacco control, and environmental health. The ALA web site provides detailed information about lung diseases, information about ALA programs and events, a list of publications, and an ALA chapter locator.

Foundation for a Smokefree America

P.O. Box 492028
Los Angeles, CA 90049-8028
Toll-Free: 800-541-7741
Phone: 310-471-4270
Fax: 310-471-0335
Web site: *http://www.anti-smoking.org*

Created by Patrick Reynolds (grandson of R. J. Reynolds), the Foundation for a Smokefree America is a nonprofit group whose mission is to educate people of all ages about smoking and tobacco use. The web sites *Anti-Smoking.org*, *NoTobacco.org*, and *TobaccoFree.org* have information about smoking and quitting tips.

Nicotine Anonymous World Services

419 Main Street, PMB #370
Huntington Beach, CA 92648
Phone: 415-750-0328
Web site: *http://www.nicotine-anonymous.org*

Nicotine Anonymous is an anonymous support group, based on a twelve-step fellowship, of people who want to live free of nicotine addiction. The web site provides: nicotine cessation and support literature in five languages, answers to frequently asked questions about nicotine addiction, and a worldwide list of meetings.

The Office on Smoking and Health (OSH)

National Center for Disease Prevention and Health Promotion/CDC
4770 Buford Highway NE
Mail Stop K-50
Atlanta, GA 30341-3724
Toll-Free: 800-CDC-1311 (800-232-1311)
Phone: 770-488-5705
Web site: *http://www.cdc.gov/tobacco*

This Centers for Disease Control and Prevention office is a division within the National Center for Chronic Disease Prevention and Health Promotion within the U.S. Department of Health and Human Services. OSH is responsible for leading and coordinating strategic efforts aimed at preventing tobacco use among youth, promoting tobacco cessation, and protecting nonsmokers from environmental tobacco smoke (ETS). The web site offers public education and information on smoking and how to stop.

QuitNet
1 Appleton Street, 4th floor
Boston, MA 02116
Phone: 617-437-1500
Fax: 617-437-9394
Web site: *http://www.quitnet.org*

QuitNet.com, Inc. is a private company operating in association with Boston University School of Public Health. It provides cutting edge, effective tobacco cessation services to people worldwide. The web site includes chat rooms, quitting guides, quitting calendars, a national directory of local smoking cessation programs, tobacco news, and personalized services like peer-to-peer support, tools to track your progress and recommend strategies, and access to online counselors. Registration is required, and some services require a fee.

The Robert Wood Johnson Foundation (RWJF)
P.O. Box 2316
Route 1 College Road East
Princeton, NJ 08543-2316
Toll-Free: 888-631-9989
Web site: *http://www.rwjf.org*

RWJF was established as a national philanthropy and is the largest U.S. foundation devoted to improving the health and health care of all Americans. In 1994 it created the program Smoke-Free Families (SFF): Innovations to Stop Smoking During and Beyond Pregnancy (*http://www.smokefreefamilies.org*).

World No Tobacco Day (WNTD)

World Health Organization
Regional Office for the Americas/Pan American Health
Organization
525 23rd Street NW
Washington, DC 20037
Phone: 202-974-3000 (Main)
Phone: 202-974-3457 (Office of Public Information)
Phone: 212-601-8245 for information about World No
Tobacco Day
Fax: 202-974-3663
Web site: *http://www.wntd.com*

The World Health Organization annually sponsors
WNTD to call attention to the seriousness of the impact of
tobacco on health. WNTD is the first and only global event
where smokers around the world unite to break free from
their dependence on tobacco. First held in 1988, and
observed annually on May 31, WNTD is the only global event
established to raise awareness of the international impact
of tobacco use and promote a tobacco-free environment.

Index